Wheelchair Yoga

Jerri Lincoln

Ralston Store Publishing
P.O. Box 4513
Durango, Colorado 81302

ISBN 978-1-938322-02-0

Disclaimer of Liability:
Not all exercise is suitable for everyone, and this or any
exercise program may result in injury. Please seek your
physician's advice before beginning any new exercise program.
The author and publisher assume no responsibility for injuries
suffered while practicing these techniques.

Printed in the USA.

Yoga feels good. You should feel good practicing yoga. If you experience any pain or discomfort, back off. You will gradually increase what you are able to do. Be kind to yourself. These gentle and easy poses work different muscles throughout your body. It is advisable to practice these yoga poses with a partner or caregiver present.

When I'm feeling tense and stressed, much of my tension goes straight into my face, especially my jaw. The next few pictures demonstrate how to relax your facial muscles. Traditional yoga poses follow.

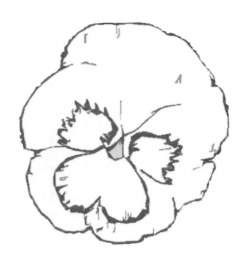

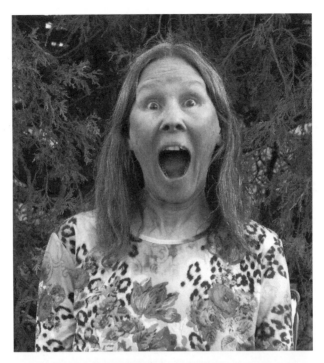

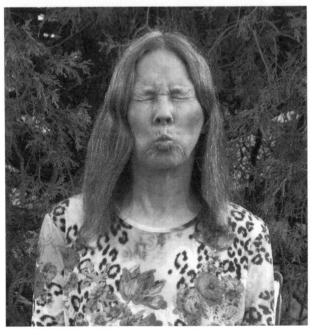

Open your mouth and eyes as wide as you can. Now close your eyes tight and press your lips together as you pucker your lips. Again, open wide and then press together. Do this five times.

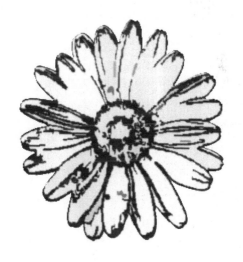

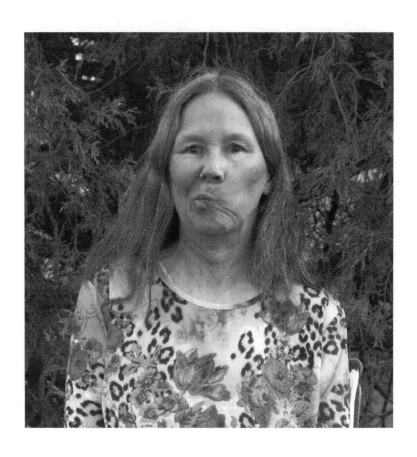

Move your lips all the way to the right, then all the way to the left. Do this five times in each direction. The more you do it, the easier it becomes.

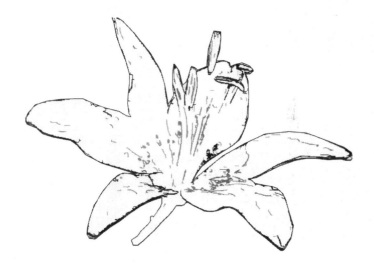

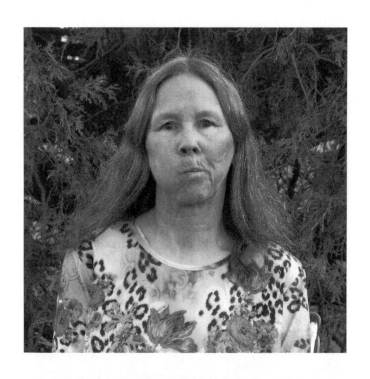

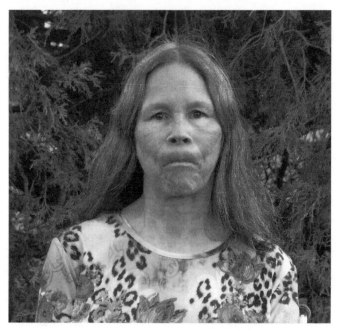

Fill your right cheek with air. Now move the air to your left cheek. Move it to your upper lip, then your lower lip. Keep doing this several times in succession. It will relax the muscles in your face.

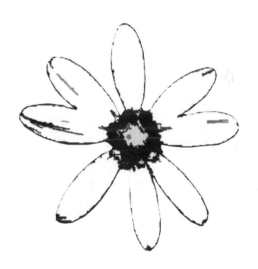

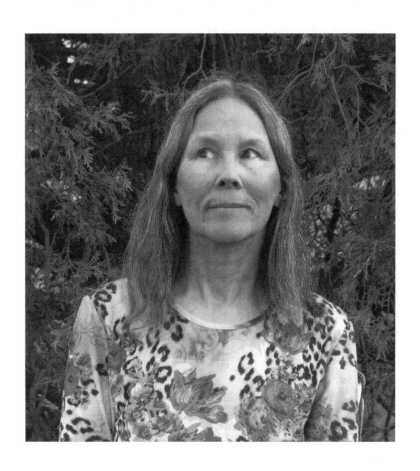

Hold your head level and look straight ahead. Keep breathing normally throughout. Without moving your head, look up to the right and then look down toward the left, back and forth ten times. Then look up toward the left and look down toward the right, back and forth ten times. Look straight up and then look straight down, back and forth ten times. This will relax your eyes.

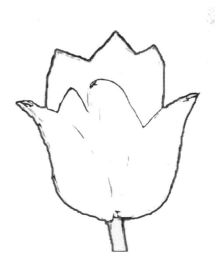

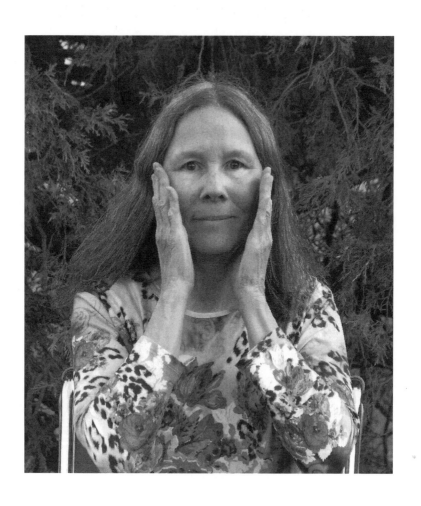

Hold your head level, raise your hands, and gently slap your cheeks one right after the other. Breathe deeply five times. This will relax your face and get the blood flowing.

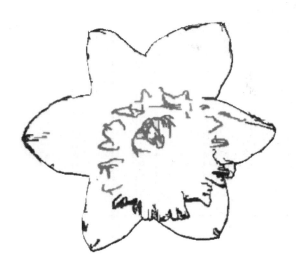

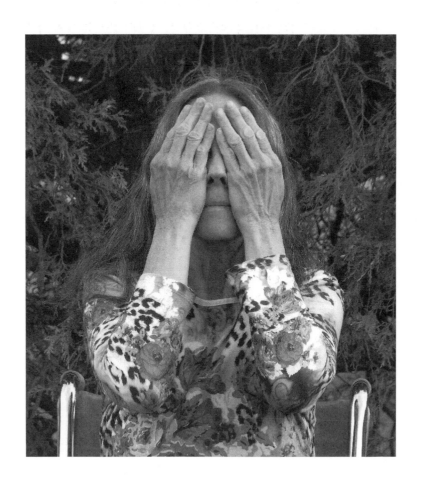

If you wear glasses, remove them. Place your hands so that the palms of your hands are covering your eyes. Breathe deeply for ten full breaths while thinking how relaxed your body is. This will relax your eyes and your body.

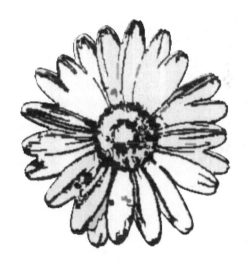

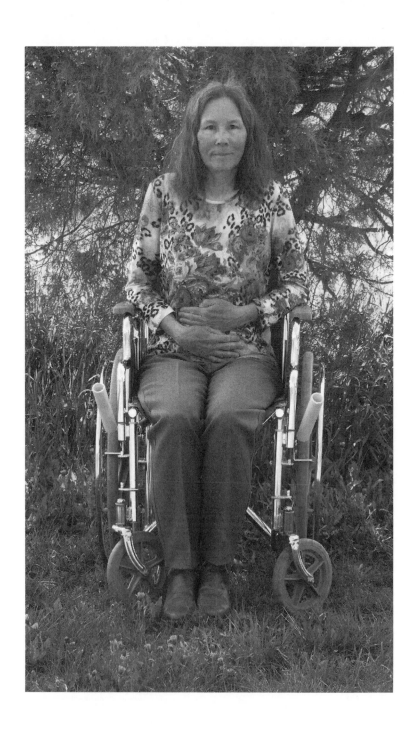

Breathing is a key part of yoga. Put your hands on your abdomen. Take a slow, deep breath through your nostrils. Feel your belly expand like a balloon inflating. As you exhale, pull in your belly like a balloon deflating. Continue taking these slow deep breaths for a few minutes.

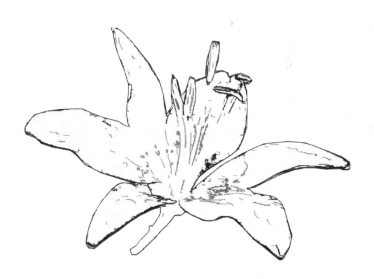

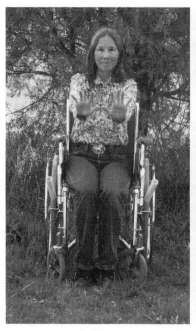 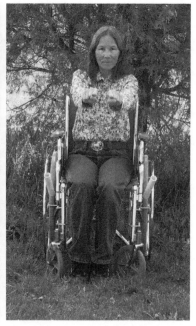

Extend both arms straight out in front of you. Stretch out and reach with your fingers as you inhale. As you exhale, clench your fingers into a fist. Repeat this pose four more times while continuing to inhale and exhale. This pose strengthens the finger and hand muscles.

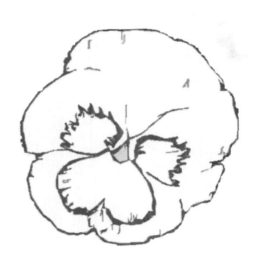

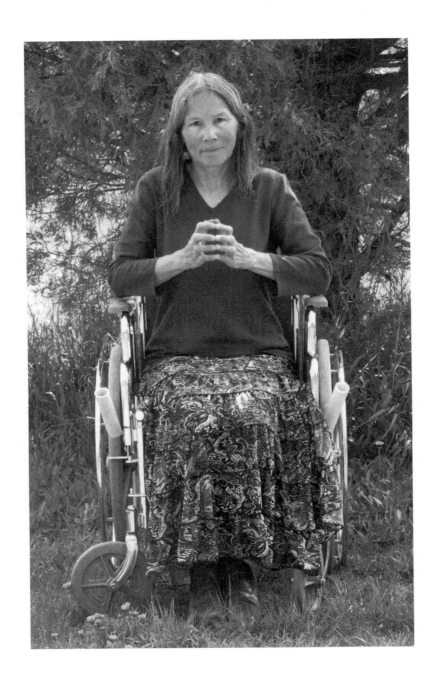

Place your fingertips together exerting some pressure. Now, like a spider doing push ups on a mirror, push your fingers against each other so the palms of your hand come closer together and then farther apart. Continue while exerting pressure. This pose strengthens the finger and hand muscles.

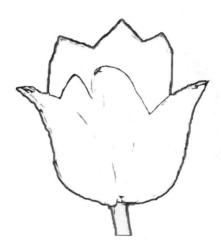

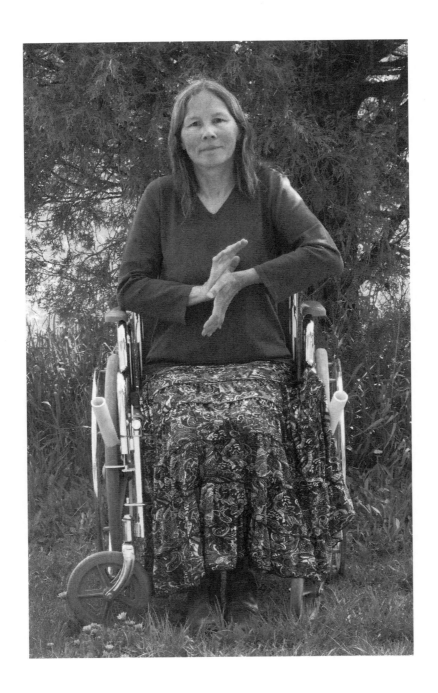

With equal pressure, press the heel of one palm against the heel of the other palm. Take one complete slow breath. First, have one hand facing up, and then the other hand. Continue breathing, and do each hand three times. This pose strengthens the hand muscles.

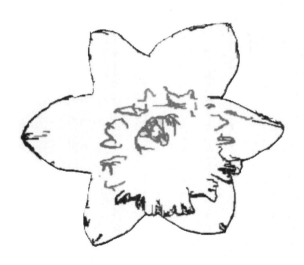

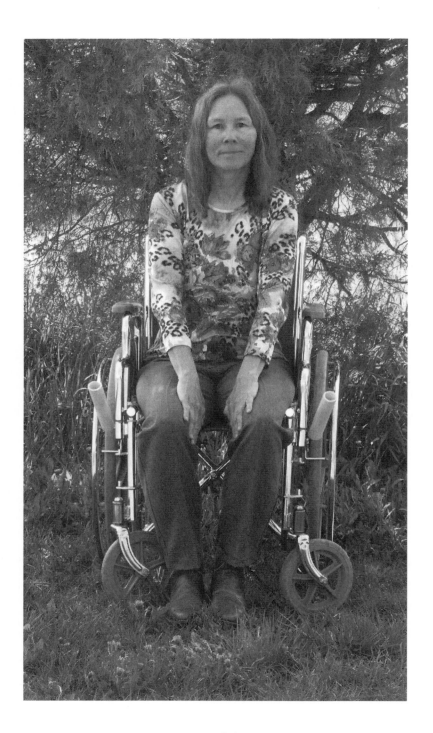

Sit with your legs slightly apart, and place your hands on the inside of your thighs, just behind the knees. Inhale as you try to press your thighs together while pushing outward with your hands. Exhale and relax. Repeat four times. This pose strengthens the thighs.

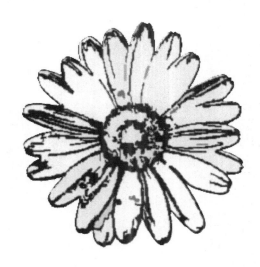

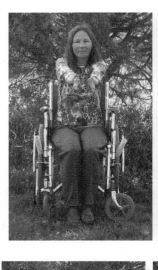 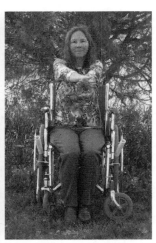

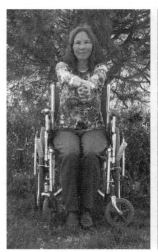 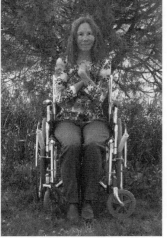

Hold your arms straight out in front of you, with your palms facing outward. Cross the right hand over the left hand, and your palms should now face each other. Interlace your fingers. Inhale as you pull your hands toward your stomach, and then up toward your chin keeping the fingers interlaced. Exhale as you stretch your arms back out, keeping the fingers interlaced. Repeat this three times remembering to inhale and exhale! Then, start again with your arms straight out in front, and this time do the entire exercise with your left hand crossed over your right hand. Repeat three times. This pose strengthens the arm muscles, calms the mind, and improves concentration.

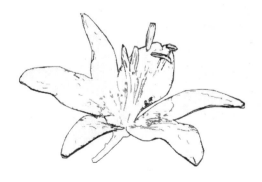

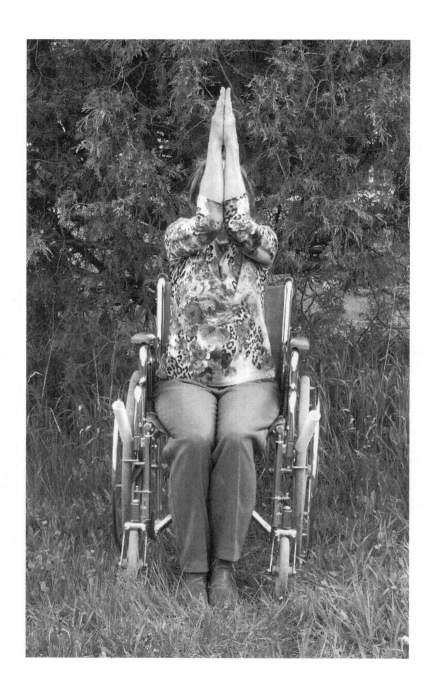

Extend your arms straight out in front of you, with the palms together and the elbows together. Keeping hands and elbows pressed together, bend at the elbow and bring your hands toward your forehead, until they are at a ninety-degree angle. Raise your arms upward as far as is comfortable. Hold the pose for five deep breaths. This pose strengthens and aligns the upper body.

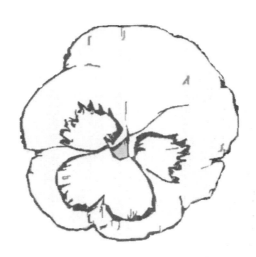

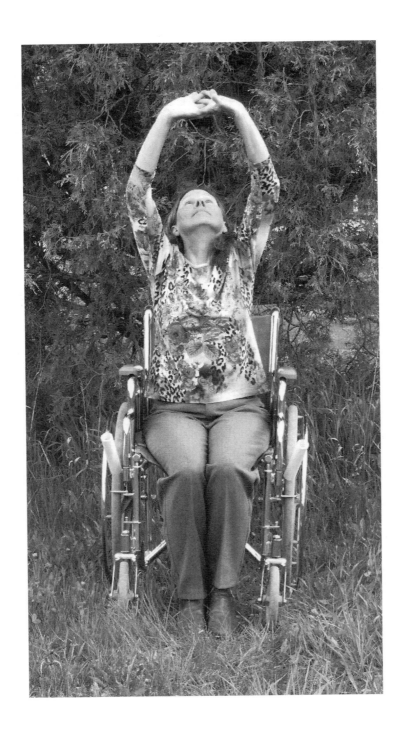

With your back straight, inhale and raise your arms over your head with your palms together. Interlace your fingers and press your palms away from your body stretching your arms and your spine upward. Tilt your head back gently to look at your hands. Exhale and take four more deep breaths. This pose stretches the belly, improves digestion, and increases circulation to the upper body and the arms, hands, and wrists.

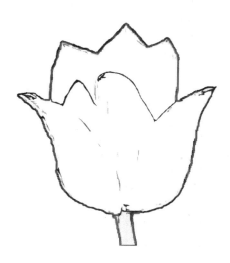

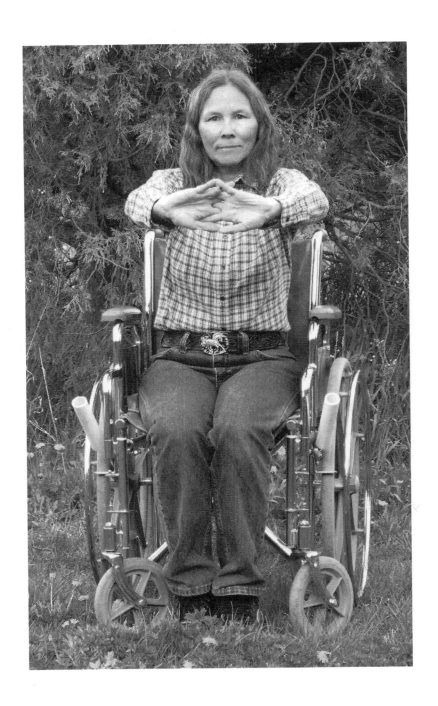

Interlace your fingers and press your palms away from your body keeping your arms at shoulder level. Hold the pose as you take five deep breaths. This pose stretches the shoulders, upper arms, and forearms.

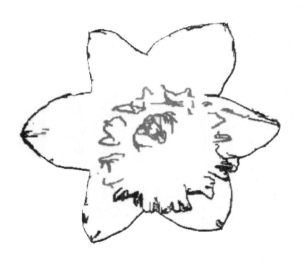

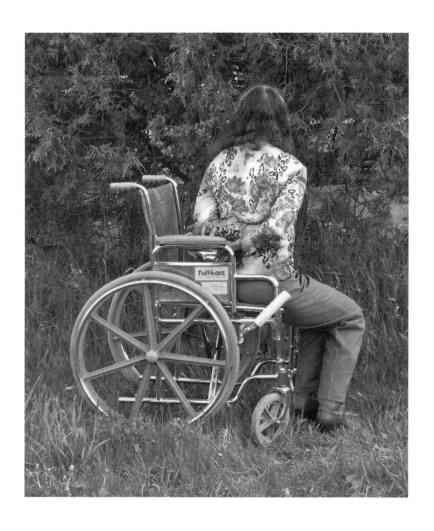

Put both hands behind your back, and clasp your arms as close as you can to the elbows. Breathe five deep breaths. Now put the opposite arm on top, and breathe five more deep breaths. This pose stretches the muscles and tendons of the arms and upper chest.

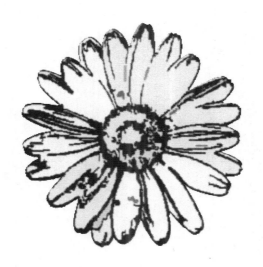

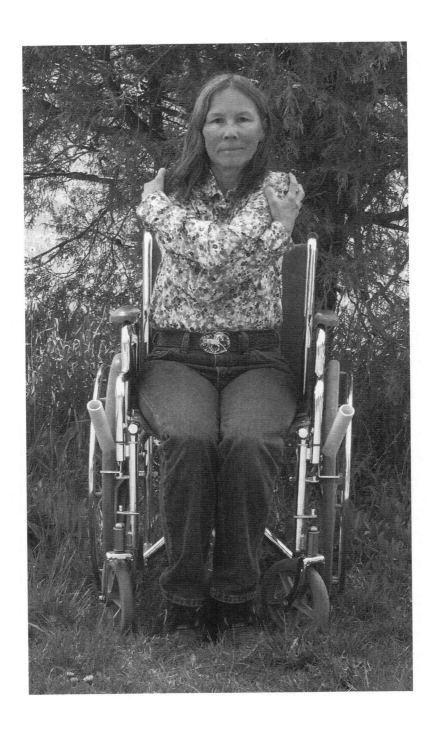

Wrap your arms around yourself in a big hug. But, not so tight that you can't breathe! Take five deep breaths. Notice which arm is on top, and switch arms. Take five more deep breaths. This pose stretches the arms and feels really good!

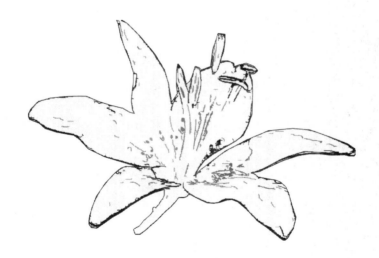

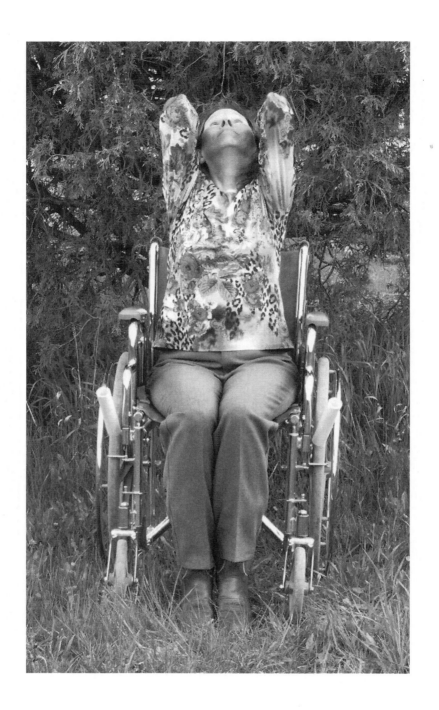

Reach behind you as if you are reaching for the back of a chair, right hand over right shoulder, and left hand over left shoulder. Your head goes back gently stretching your neck and you should have a slight arch to your back. Breathe deeply for five breaths. This pose increases flexibility in the back.

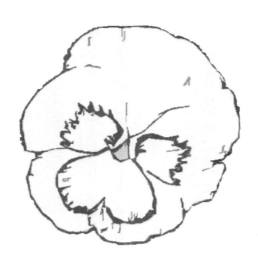

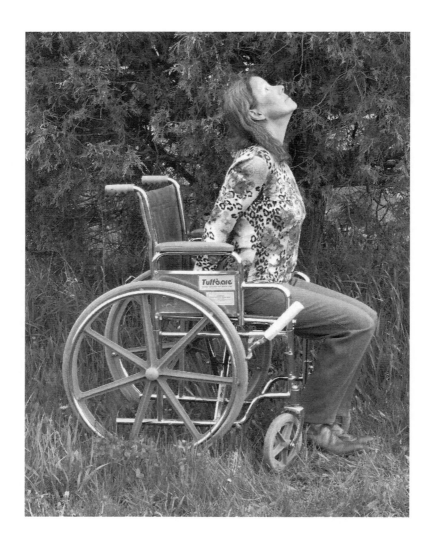

Place your hands behind you on the seat. Inhale and lift your chest upward as you look upward. Continue breathing five deep breaths. This pose increases flexibility in the back and shoulders.

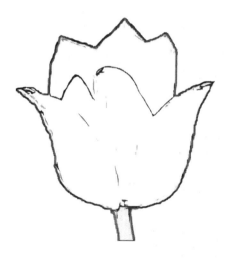

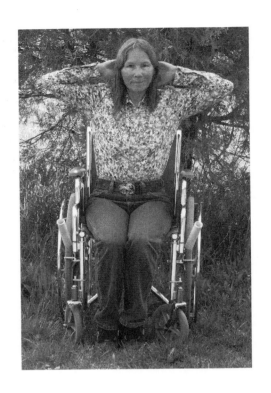

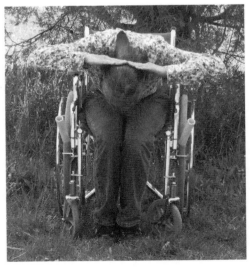

Put your hands gently behind your head, fingers barely touching, not pushing on your head. Come forward slowly into a forward bend, without putting any pressure on your head. Breathe five deep breaths, and then come up slowly one vertebra at a time. This pose stretches the arms, the hips, and the back.

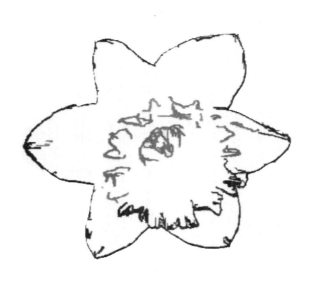

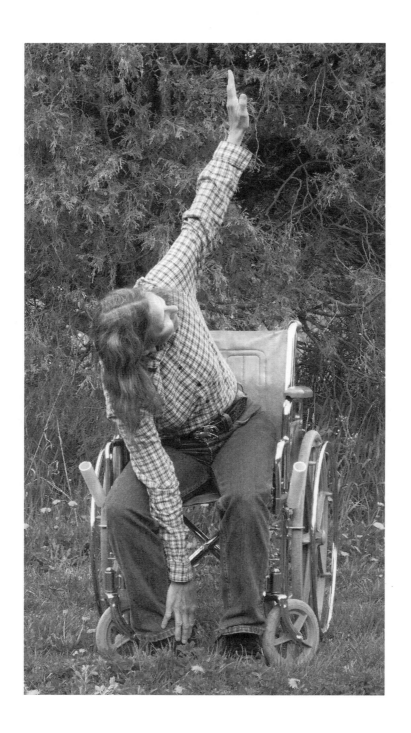

Slightly separate your legs. As you reach down with your right hand to the inside of your right ankle, raise your left arm up and look up. Breathe five deep breaths and come back to center. Then, reach down with your left hand to the inside of your left ankle, and raise your left arm up and look up. Breathe five deep breaths before you come back to center. This pose stretches the arms, back, and shoulders.

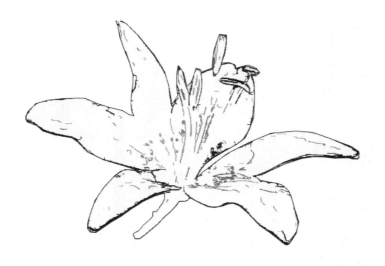

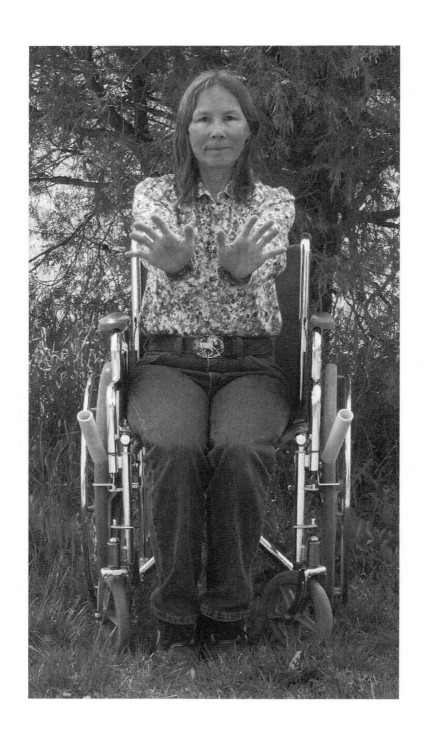

Stretch your arms straight out in front of you. Flex your wrists up and down, and then rotate them first in one direction and then the other. This pose loosens and lubricates the joints.

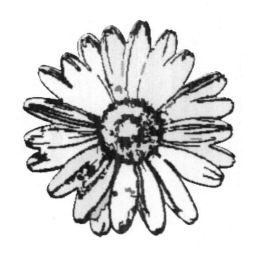

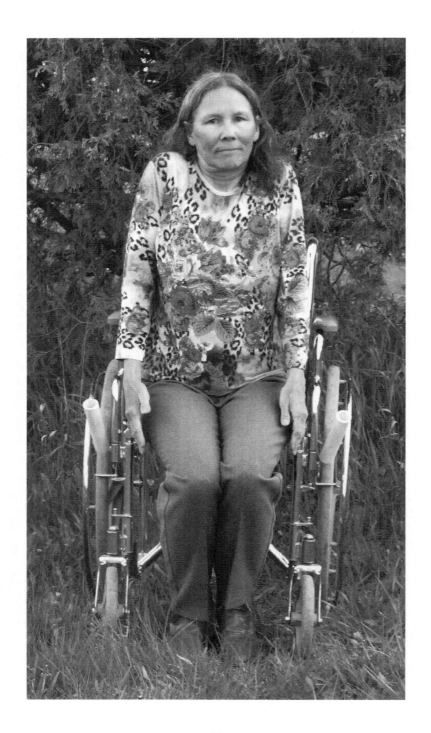

Sit up straight. Inhale as you raise your shoulders toward your ears. Exhale, and let them drop back down. Repeat five times. This pose strengthens the shoulder area, and relieves tension in the neck and shoulders.

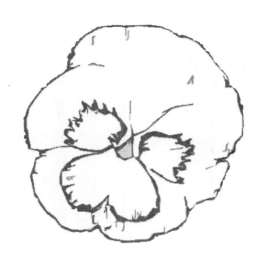

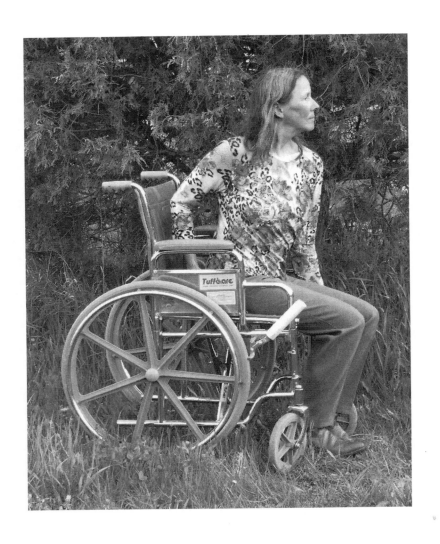

With your back straight, and looking straight ahead, roll one shoulder forward and then the other, like walking with your shoulders. Do each shoulder five times, and then reverse the direction by rolling each shoulder backward five times, like walking backward. This pose strengthens the shoulders, and relieves tension.

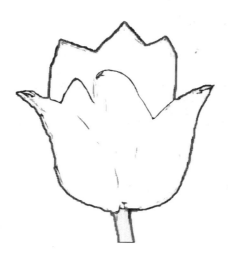

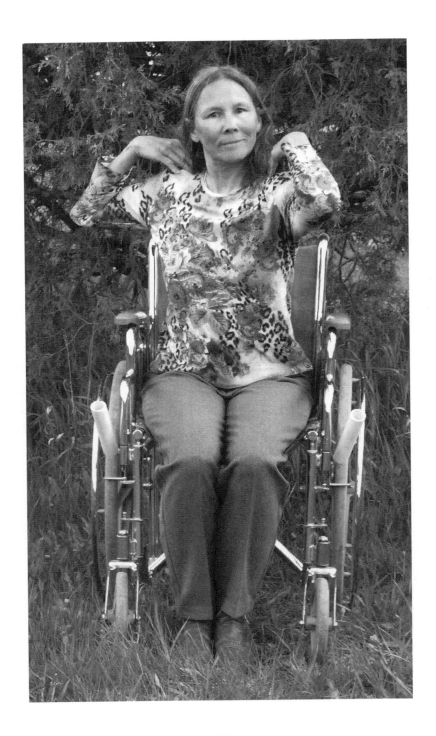

Place your right hand on your right shoulder, and your left hand on your left shoulder. Now begin making swimming-like movements, by moving your elbow forward and then around, first one elbow and then the other. Repeat five times, and then reverse direction by moving your elbow back and then around. Repeat five times. This pose strengthens the shoulders, and releases tension in the shoulder and upper back.

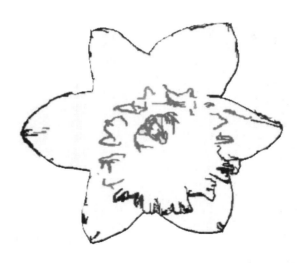

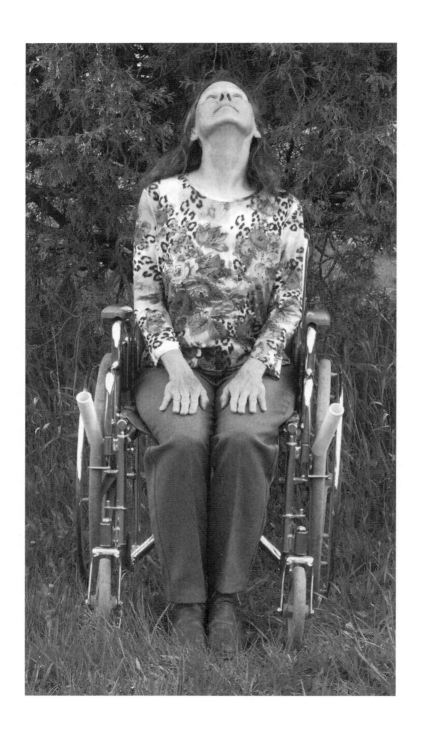

Take a deep breath. With your back straight, and looking straight ahead, on the exhale tilt your head forward so your chin goes toward your chest. Inhale back up. Repeat two more times. On the next exhale, lift your chin and tilt your head backward toward your back. Inhale back up, and repeat two more times. On the next exhale, bring your right ear toward your shoulder. Inhale back up, and repeat two more times. Next exhale, bring your left ear toward your shoulder. Inhale back up, and repeat two more times. Finally, starting at the chin toward chest position, move your head toward the right, then the back, then the left, then the chest again, doing neck circles. Do the circle twice in each direction. This pose creates greater flexibility and range of motion in the neck.

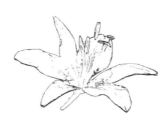

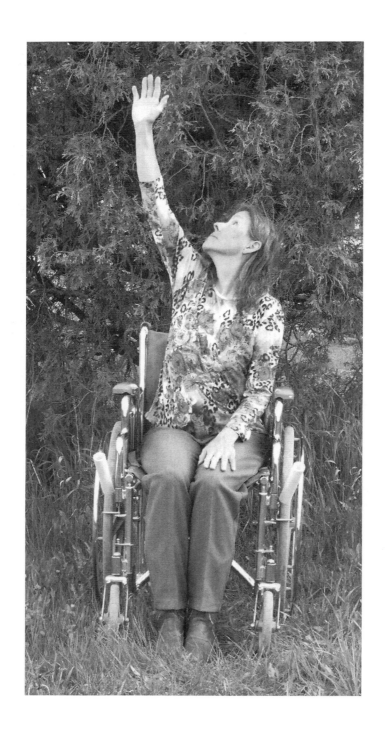

Keeping your back straight, inhale as you raise one arm over your head, turning your head to look up at it. Exhale and bring the arm back down. Inhale as you raise the other arm over your head, turning your head to look up at it. Exhale and bring the arm back down. Raise each arm four more times. This pose lengthens and strengthens the back, and strengthens the shoulders.

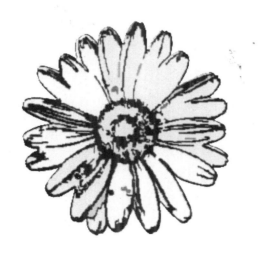

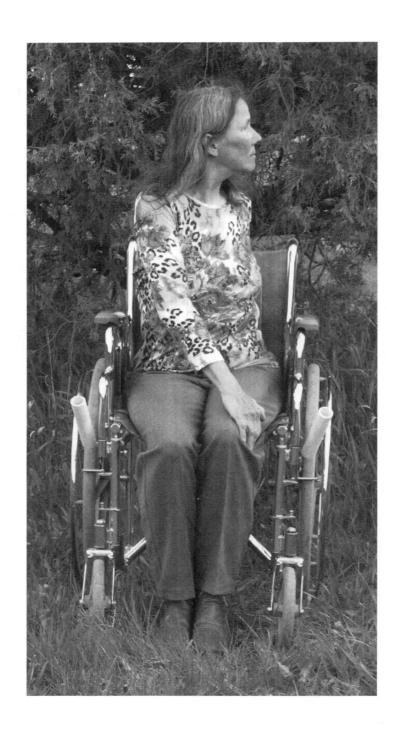

Put your left hand on your right knee.
With your knees facing forward, turn
your body to the right and look right.
Take five deep breaths. Come slowly
back to center. Put your right hand on
your left knee. With your knees still
facing forward, turn your body to the
left and look left. Take five more
deep breaths. This pose stretches the
back, the shoulders, and the hips.

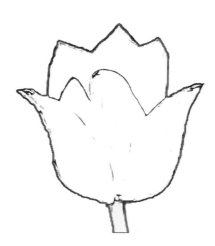

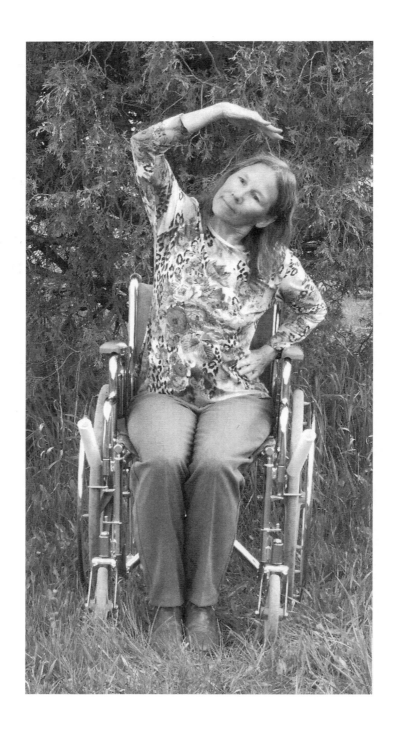

Raise your right arm straight up, and put your left hand on your left hip. Bend toward the left, bringing your right hand over your head. Hold for five breaths. Come back to center and lower your arm. Raise your left arm straight up, and put your right hand on your right hip. Bend toward the right, bringing your left hand over your head. Hold for five breaths. This pose strengthens the spine, the neck, and the arms.

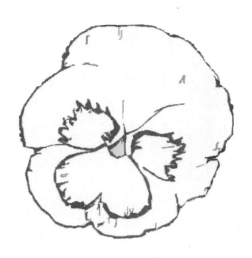

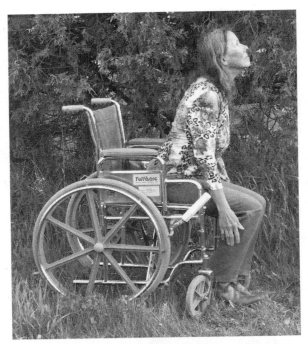

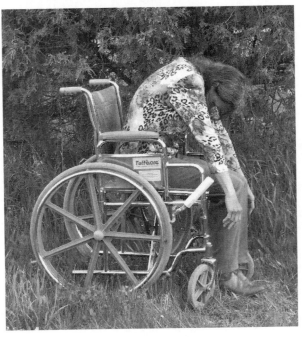

Start with your back straight and your hands on your knees. Slowly inhale and lift your chest up and forward, creating a slight arch in your back while your head faces forward and slightly up. Slowly exhale while rounding your back, pulling in your belly, and tucking your chin into your chest. Repeat this slowly five times. These two poses increase spinal flexibility and abdominal strength.

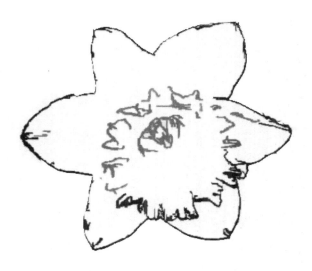

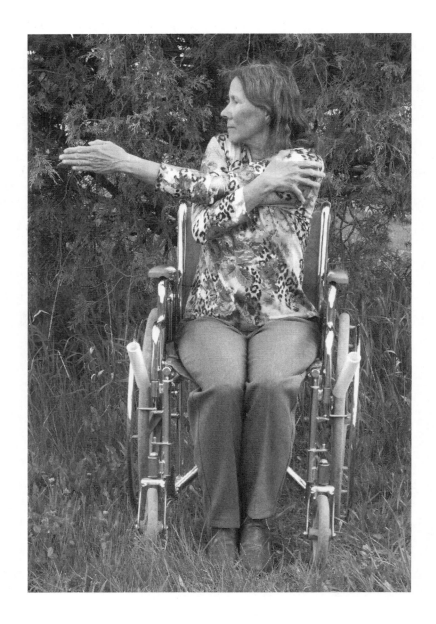

Reach straight out in front of you with your right arm, while stretching your fingers. Move your arm slowly to the left. Take your left hand and put it on your right upper arm, and pull it in toward your chest. Hold for five deep breaths. Release your right arm. Now, reach straight out in front of you with your left arm, while stretching your fingers. Move your arm slowly to the right. Take your right hand and put it on your left upper arm, and pull it in toward your chest. Hold for five deep breaths. This is a good stretch for your shoulders.

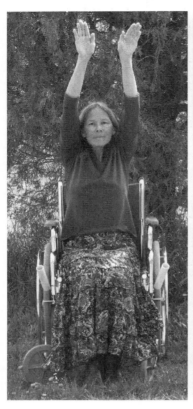

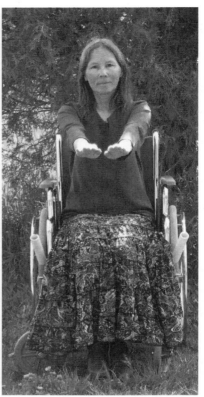

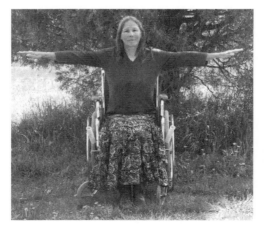

Breathe in as you raise your arms straight up over your head. Exhale as you lower your arms so that they are straight out in front of you. Take another deep breath as you extend your arms to your sides and then slowly exhale. Feel the stretch from your shoulders and upper back to the tips of your fingers. Bring your arms back in front of you, and then repeat movements four times. This is a good stretch for arms and shoulders.

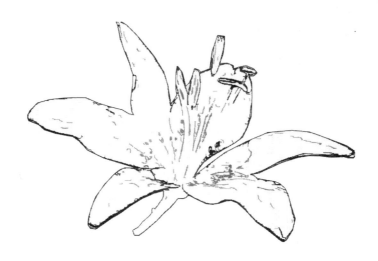

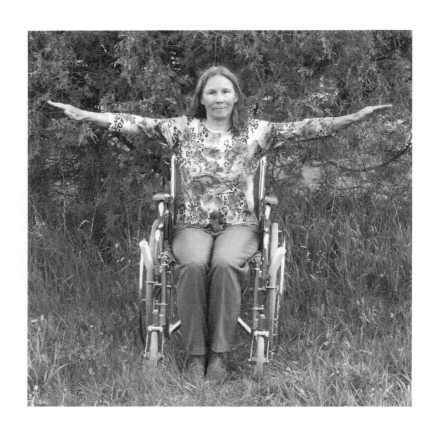

Stretch your arms out to your sides.
Rotate your arms forward ten times in
large circles. Reverse direction for
ten more times. This pose strengthens
the shoulders and upper arms.

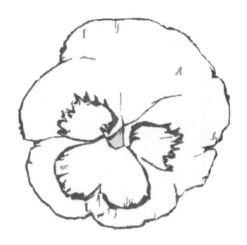

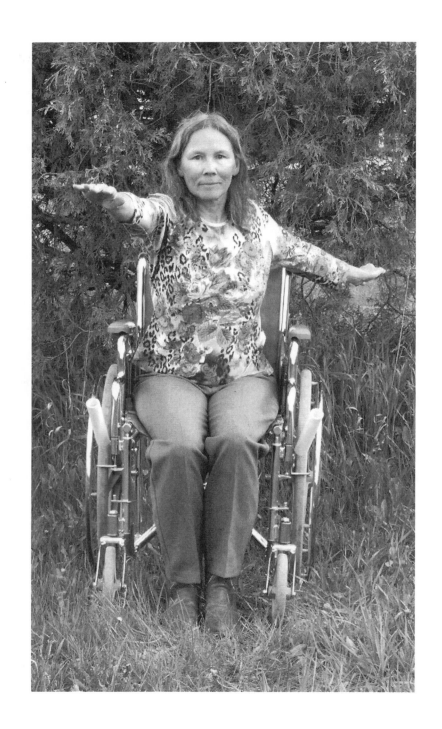

"Swim" with the crawl stroke ten times for each arm. Then reverse and do the "back stroke" ten times for each arm. This exercise is good for your arms and upper body.

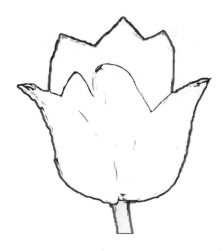

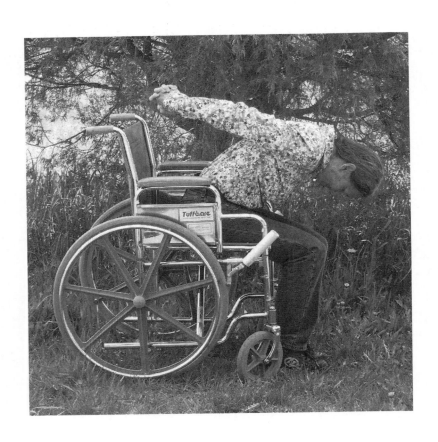

Reach both arms behind your back and interlace your fingers. Now lean forward and raise your arms as high as they will comfortably go. Take five slow deep breaths. This pose stretches the muscles in the chest and the shoulders.

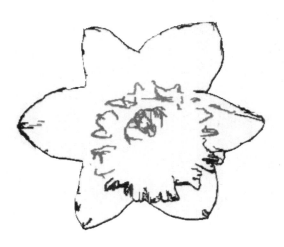

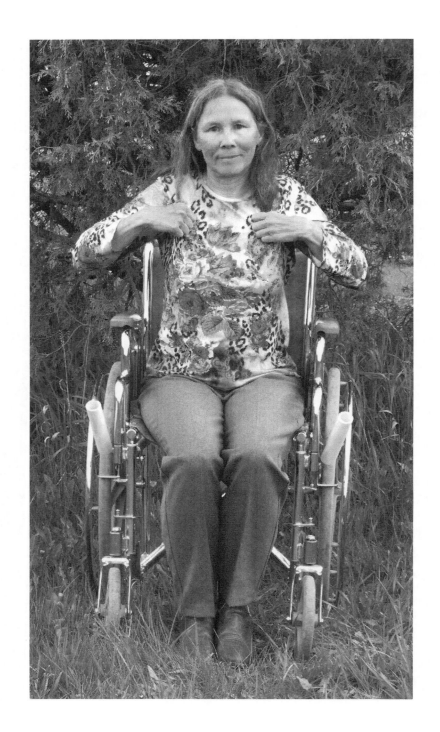

Put your thumbs in your armpits, and flap your arms energetically! This pose releases tension in the shoulders.

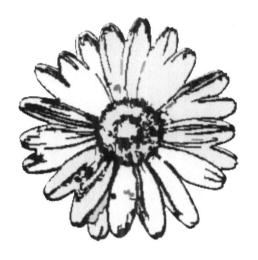

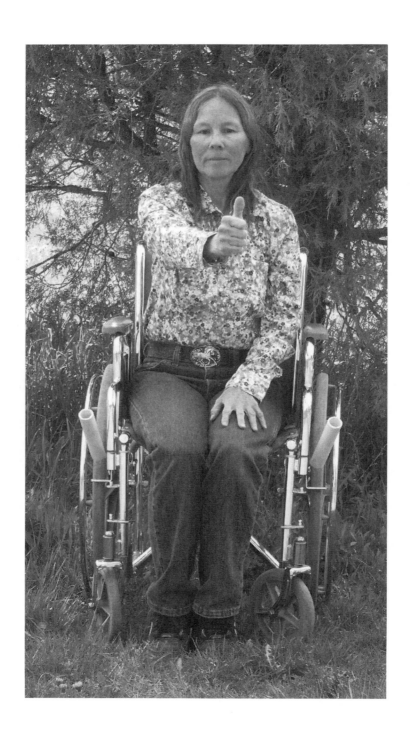

Reach out in front of you with your right hand, thumb up. Move it slightly left so it is in the center of your body. Start by moving your thumb up to the left, and draw sideways figure eights. Make sure that the thumb crosses the midline of your body. Keep going to make five eights, and then do the same thing five times with your left hand, moving up to the right. Follow your thumb with your eyes, but don't move your head. This pose balances the two hemispheres of the brain.

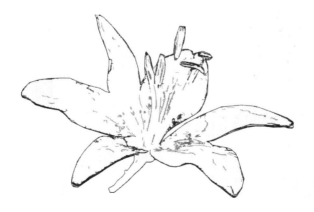

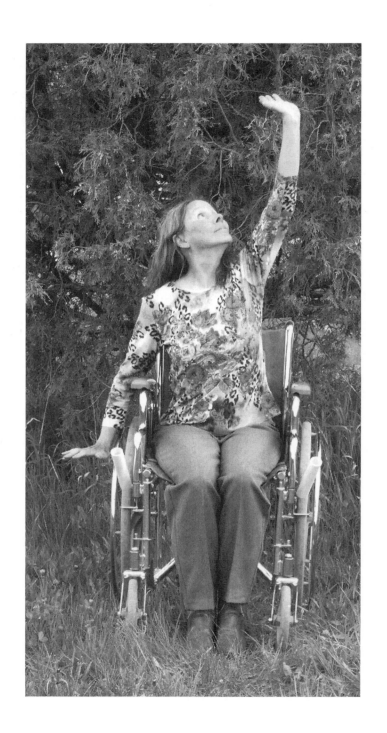

Raise your right arm and flatten your hand as if you are holding up the sky. Lower your left arm and flatten your hand as if you are holding down the earth. Look at the upward arm. Feel the stretch. Take several breaths and then repeat with the left arm raised, and the right arm down. Again, look at the upward arm. This pose strengthens the shoulders and the back muscles.

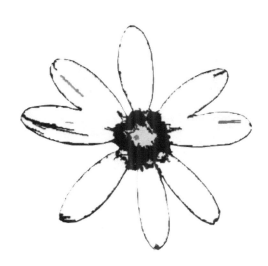

Now for something different! Do the next twelve poses in a flowing sequence one right after the other like a dance. This group of poses relieves tension and enhances circulation.

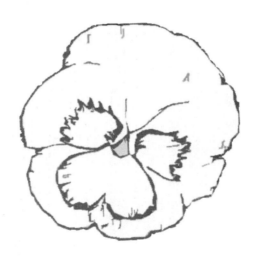

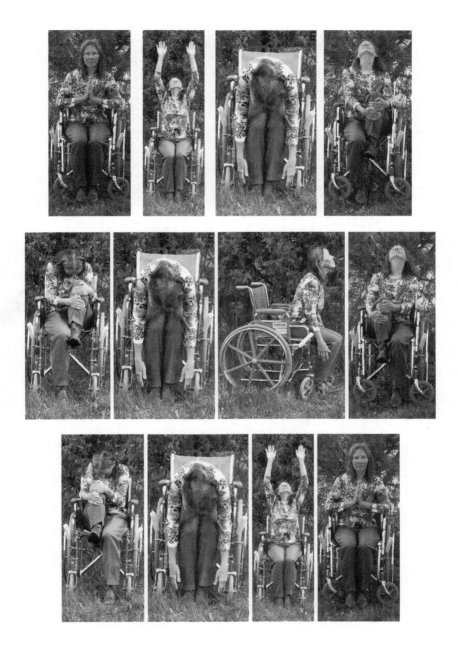

Turn to the next page for directions.

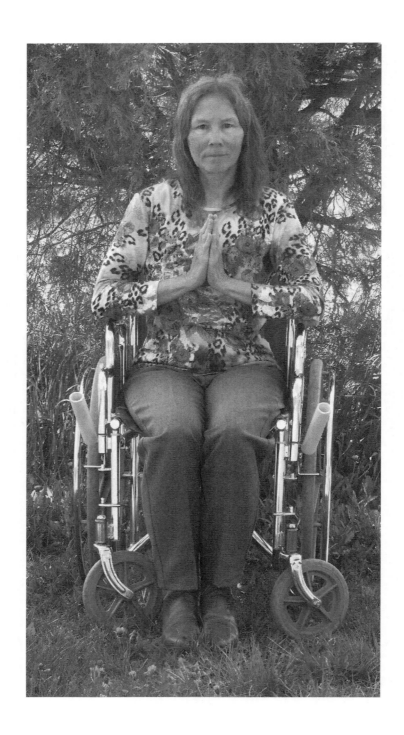

Hands to your heart, with palms together.

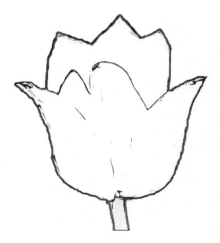

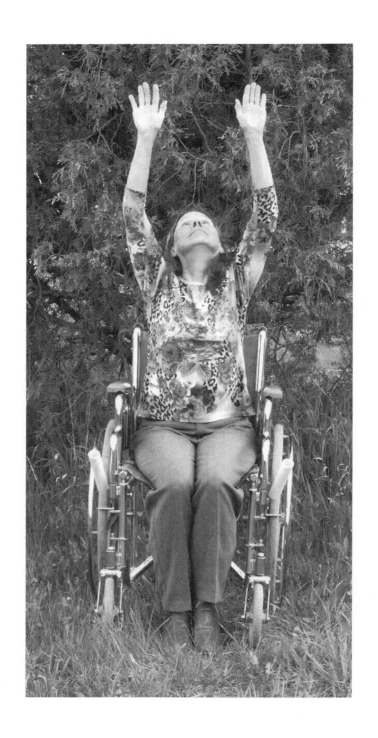

Inhale and reach upward with your arms, looking up, and arching your back.

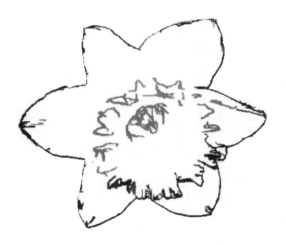

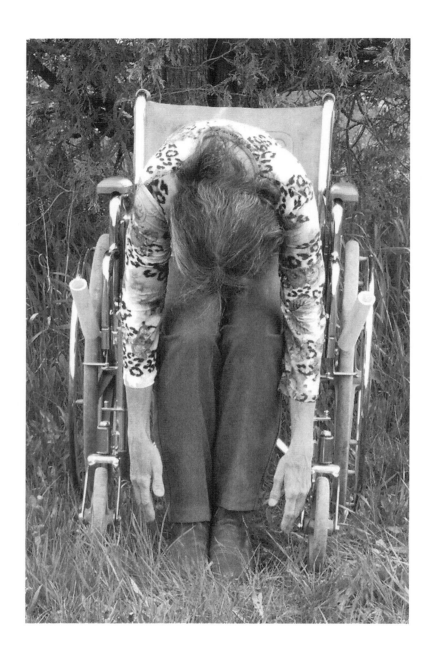

Exhale, and bend forward slowly,
with your hands beside your feet.

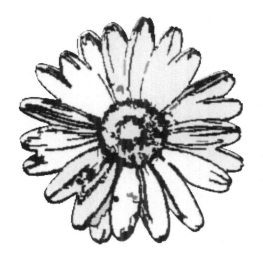

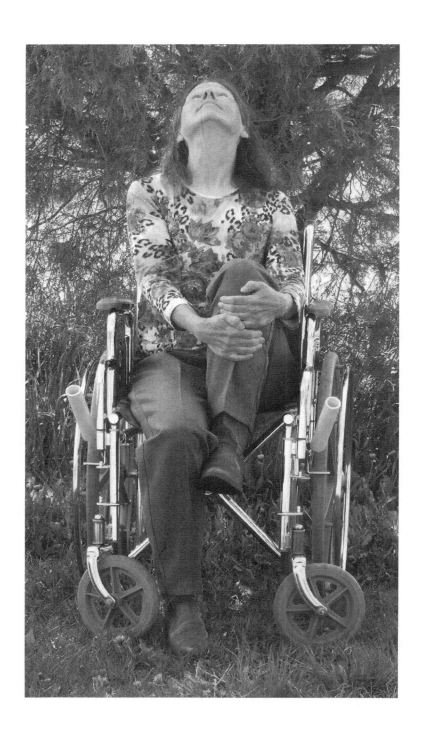

Inhale, and pull your left knee into your chest. Look upward, and have your back slightly arched.

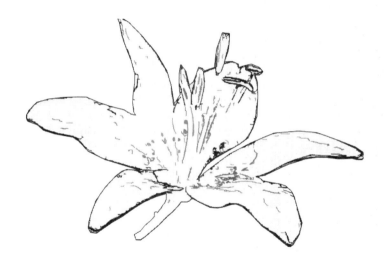

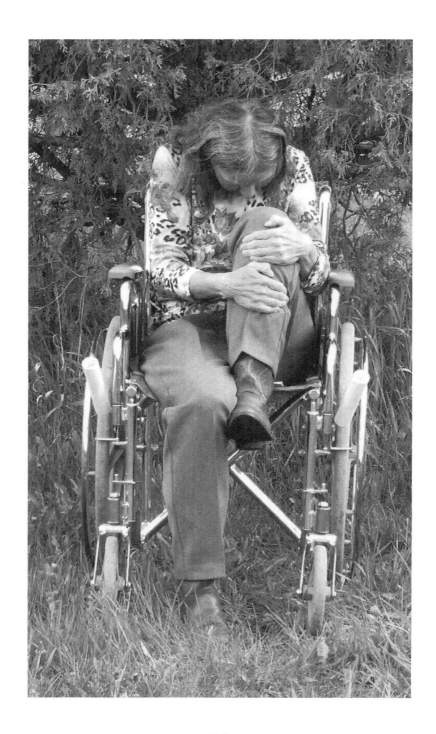

Start to exhale as you bring your chin to your chest and your forehead to your knee.

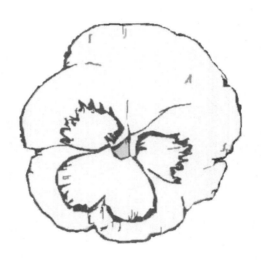

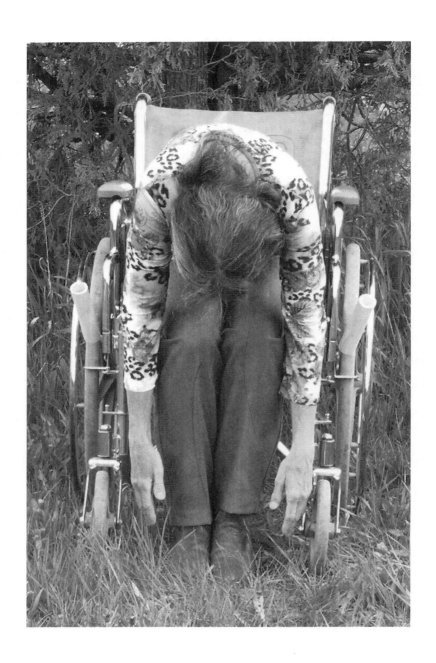

Finish your exhale as you bend forward slowly, with your hands beside your feet.

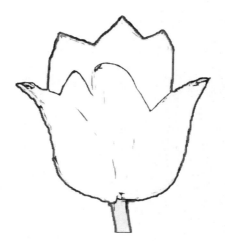

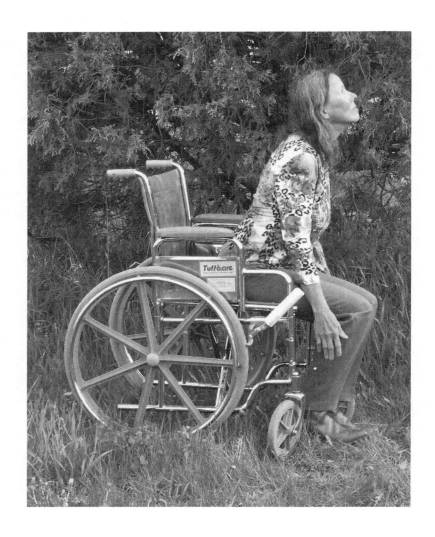

Start to inhale as you arch your back and neck, with your hands down by your legs.

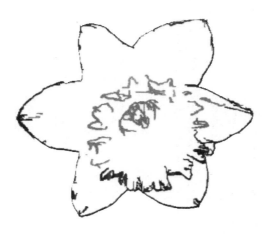

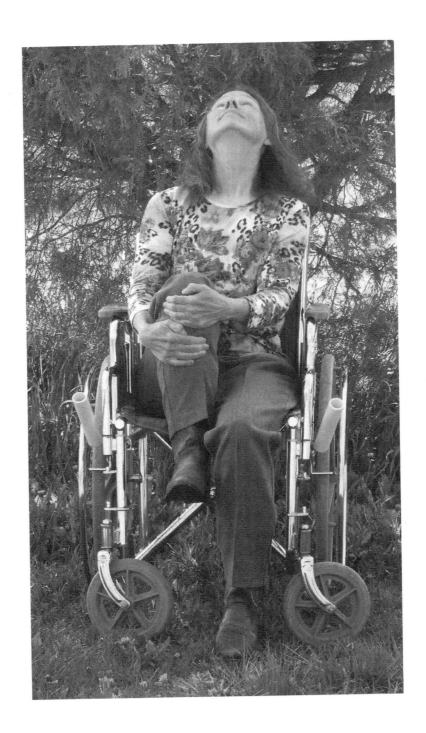

Complete your inhale as you pull your right knee toward your chest. Look upward and have your back slightly arched.

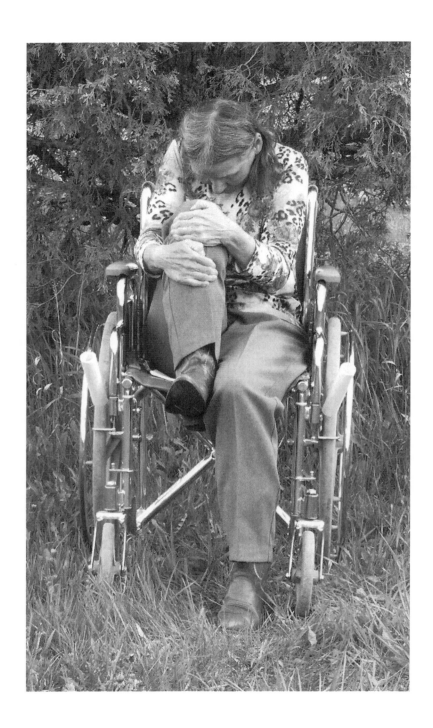

Start to exhale as you bring your chin to your chest and your forehead toward your knee.

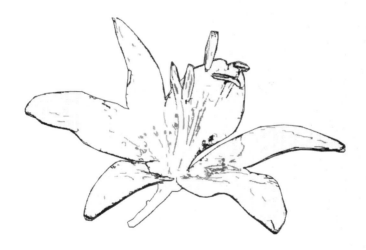

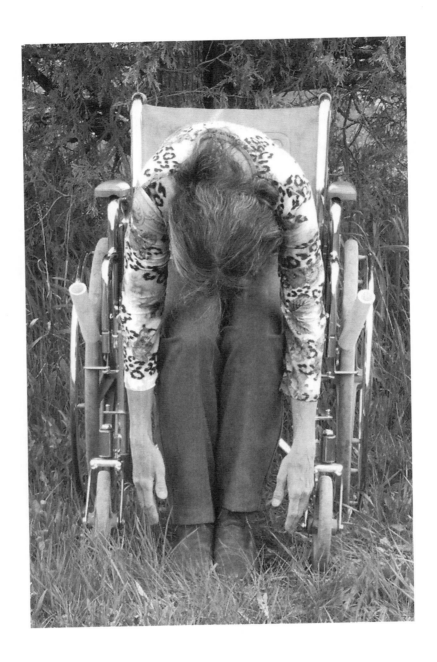

Finish your exhale as you bend
forward slowly, with your hands
beside your feet.

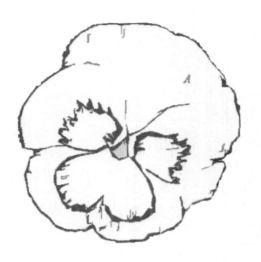

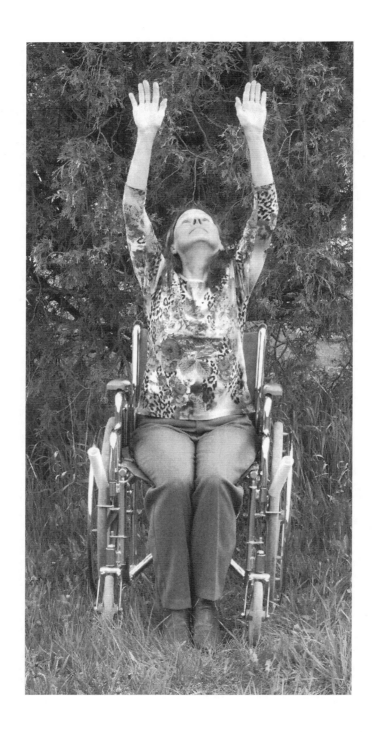

Inhale and reach upward with your arms, looking up, and arching your back.

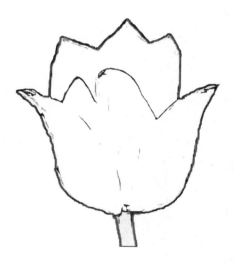

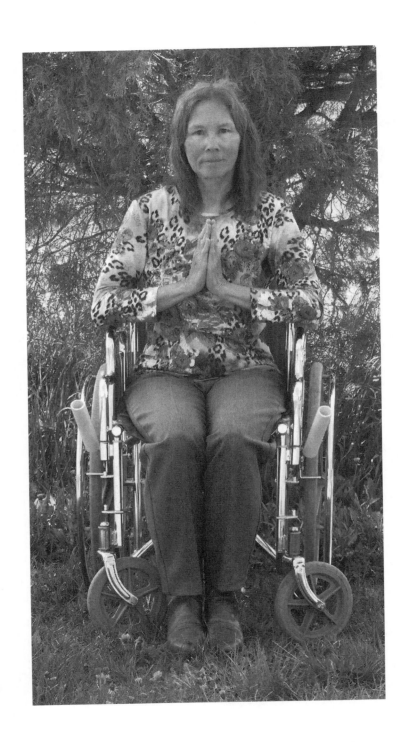

Exhale. Hands to your heart, with palms together.

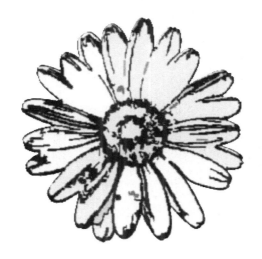

About the Author

Jerri Lincoln was certified to teach yoga and meditation at the Chopra Center in Carlsbad, California. She has written several specialized yoga books including one on therapeutic riding. Twenty-five per cent of proceeds from that book go to Cadence Therapeutic Riding Center in Durango, Colorado.